Maximum Energy: 5 tips to increasing your energy and reducing fatigue

Disclaimer and Terms of Use: Effort has been made to ensure that the information in this book is accurate and complete, however, the author and the publisher do not warrant the accuracy of the information, text and graphics contained within the book due to the rapidly changing nature of science, research, known and unknown facts and internet. The Author and the publisher do not hold any responsibility for errors, omissions or contrary interpretation of the subject matter herein. This book is presented solely for motivational and informational purposes only.

Table of Contents

ABSTRACT

While technically the famous adage goes- "You are only as old as you actually feel", how about replacing 'old' with 'tired', 'drained' and 'rundown'? When you realize you have barely copped a few Z's last night, playing hooky (from the family, from the job and from life) doesn't really sound like an amusing idea! And with those energy levels falling into a red zone, caffeine seems to be the only quick fix Band-Aid. Well, there's good news. If fatigue is something that now seems to be like a common feeling to you, you need help! Making a few tweaks here and there in your lifestyle and eating habits can reduce the problem significantly. This report encompasses the whole gamut of tried and tested tips to combat fatigue and jazz up your life by boosting energy.

It consists of five sections. The first part deals with eight essential foods which when incorporated into your diet can bolster your energy and get you on your foot. The second section concerns itself with the changes one can make in his eating habits, to eliminate any chances of falling prey to the ogre named fatigue. This report explicates the relationship between sleeping habits and energy slumps, and also some little sleep-pattern modifications in the third section. Finally, people can discover the tips to beat lethargy with a few lifestyle changes and psychological training in the last two sections.

INTRODUCTION

Fatigue, a close relative of lethargy, exhaustion, listlessness and tiredness is a state (mental or physical) of feeling weak or tired. It is a common complaint among working employees that suddenly in the third quarter of the day, a violent or vice grip squeezes their entire energy, engulfing them and putting them into a state of dead tiredness. The steep drop in energy level hits you like a fury, virtually paralyzing your body and making you feel dead on your feet. Whether fatigue is an indication of physical exertion, emotional stress, improper eating habits, lack of sleep or boredom, it can be traced to at least one of your routines or habits. Dr. Jacob Teitelbaum suggests that we are facing a crisis of energy of historical proportions. In fact, a recent report conducted by USDA revealed that women who are in their 30's consume about 165 milligrams of caffeine each day and by the age of 50, the figure leaps to 225.

That said it's not a name of game to swig those crazily canned concoctions. Nor is it necessary to scrap your everyday Starbucks (the antioxidants are actually good for health). But what needs to go on exile is your habit of relying on 7-8 cups of caffeine/ energy drinks to keep you going through the day. So instead of applying a bandage on exhaustion, beat fatigue forever and for real by taking cues from these out-of-the-box tips.

Reversing fatigue with food

Striving to stay zippy through the day can be an ordeal. And if you face the reality, exercising it away is not all that brings a revolution; what you feed those muscles with plays an equally significant role. To stay healthy and energetic, you need to step out of your several- hours- a-day gym schedule and step into your kitchen. Here is a list of the top eleven super foods that help reduce fatigue naturally-

- **Lentils:** Though tiny, yet these mighty legumes teem with a perfect combination of slow digestive proteins, fiber and complex carbohydrates to make a distinctive staple for the non vegetarians as well as vegans. Half a cup of these cooked legumes furnishes you with more protein than contained in an egg and almost a quarter more of your daily fiber dose. Their ability to get cooked without soaking makes them an efficient food for those who can't find time to adjust a cooking routine in their daily grinding.

- **Melons:** Apart from being an explosive source of vitamins and energizing minerals, melons like watermelon, cantaloupe and honeydew are composed of 90% water by weight and keep you hydrated to combat fatigue. Even a slight amount of dehydration in human body culminates in an overall lowering of energy levels and mood swings. Diced cantaloupe, melon salad or a cup of juice extracted from watermelon as a hydrating morning snack is sufficient to boost your spirits internally and physically.

- **Icelandic Yogurt:** A thick and creamy concoction as it is, Icelandic Yogurt gives its Greek counterpart a hard time. The fat content is the only straddling line between the two yogurts. While adding fat is just a choice in Greek yogurts, Icelandic yogurts are known for being fat-free. It is made from non-fatty milk and is known to be a natural energy supplement.

- **Farmer's Cheese:** Butter, cream cheese and margarine are foods that are favorable only if you wish to add a few extra layers of flab to your stomach. So it's time to ditch those fat filled foods and add some protein to the morning meals. Farmer's Cheese is manufactured using the milk of cows, sheep and goats, hence understandable rich with proteins and other nutrients. Statistically speaking, a couple of tablespoons of this cheese are enough to deliver four grams of protein while adding only 40 calories and 2.5 grams of fat.

- **Walnuts:** When we speak of foods that reduce fatigue, walnuts cannot just escape the notice. It is one of the rarely found melatonin sources- a crucial hormone, naturally produced by human body once the sun sets in evening. Its modus operandi incorporates - regulating body clock- making your eyes drowsy- helping you sleep soundly- and eventually upping your energy levels and refreshing your system in the morning. The only loophole being, as your hair gets greyer, the body cannot produce melatonin in the desired quantity; which is why a supplement like walnuts is necessary. Walnuts work best when taken as a night snack or sprinkled over fresh salad and fruit smoothies.

- **Crabs:** Crabs are not only a delicious and super-lean source of proteins, but they also teem with Vitamin B-12 to balance your mood and fight your war against listlessness. Vitamin B-12 supplements are also an excellent way to keep the red blood cells healthy and stable which in turn pumps more oxygen to the brain, letting us think clearly, positively and feel energized. It is also naturally found in chicken, meat and fish.
- **Brown Rice:** Besides being packed with carbohydrates, brown rice is a top notch source of magnesium. A drop in magnesium level may hinder with metabolism of the body and create a feeling of drowsiness and tiredness. Half a cup of brown rice should suffice for the magnesium requirement in a human body.
- **Green Tea:** It's a common substitute for the caffeine contained in coffee, green tea is good news for coffee addicts. Its amino acid rich content rejuvenates the body and makes you feel revitalized while barring the jitters from coffee. This compound is highly recommended to protect oneself from

energy robbing illnesses such as cold and common flu. Consume green tea twice on a daily basis for effective results.

Dietary suggestions to boost energy

It's not just 'what', but also 'how' and 'when' that matters when it comes to eating habits. Professional dieticians assert that taking care of your stomach and following a recommended diet in proper way is vital to stay breezy and energetic the entire day! So drop those energy shots right away and stick to the suggestions mentioned below-

- **Drink your way to an energetic day:** As it has been long established by now, a dehydrated body is of no use more than a bicycle's peddle to a wheelchair. Lack of body fluids zaps your energy and causes impairment in physical performance. Drink plenty of water before and after your meals to stay invigorated.

- **Be cautious of caffeine intake:** A cup or two of caffeinated drinks such as coffee, cola or tea per day works in your favor and creates mental alertness. However, too much of something is always harmful. People with heavy caffeine addiction tend to perform poorly and are prone to irritability and anxiety.

- **Eat before you leave:** Morning meals are crucial to a working human body. Having breakfast elevates metabolism rates and furnishes your body with energy to burn. Choose your meal that is rich in carbohydrates like wholegrain bread and cereals.

- **Avoid skipping meals:** Skipping is good, only if it's done with a rope, not on your meals. Blood sugar takes a dip when the body does not receive food for long. Consider your body as a car and your meal as the fuel. No device can function properly without the necessary fuel.

- **Do not overeat:** Large meals tend to drain the energy out of a human body. Instead of relying on three large meals, try five or six small meals to spread the kilojoules intake evenly. Not only does it result in constant energy and insulin levels, but also aids in burning extra fat.

Improving sleeping habits to overcome fatigue

Sleep deprivation is often pointed out as a key factor in causing fatigue and energy deficiency. However, by modifying our sleep patterns, we can not only combat but also win this race. Here are a handful of tips-

- **Sleep enough:** A minimum of eight hours sleep is recommended to stay young and fresh. Lack of sleep results in frustration, low energy level and poor performance throughout the day.
- **Fix your sleep time:** A Sunday is no excuse to stay awake late night and watch your favorite TV show. Set your body clock by going to bed the same time. An irregular schedule would only aggravate insomnia and increase fatigue.
- **Limit caffeine:** Eating or drinking too much caffeine in evening allows sleep to elude you and make you insomniac. To change sleep cycles in a day, inhibit yourself from eating 15-16 hours before going to bed.
- **Relax:** The most commonly found reason of sleep deprivation is fretting about several problems while trying to sleep. Experiment with a gamut of relaxation techniques available on the internet and focus on breathing patterns to soothe your senses.
- **Power naps:** You were all good in the morning, but now suddenly it seems you're about to pass out. Do not attempt pulling off a Rip Van Winkle, instead take a midday nap. The optimal amount is ten to twenty minutes of midday sleep to avoid throwing off your night's sleep.

- **Say no to sleeping pills:** No matter how much tempting those little dolls look on your table, avoid sleeping pills as they are not a long term answer to insomnia.

Lifestyle suggestions for an energetic morning

As they rightly say, "A little prevention is far better than cure", a bit of watching- the- steps is vital to ward off the major triggering factors of fatigue. Whether it's your droopy eyes, frustrated mood or tiredness, the following tweaks in your daily routine might help to trim the exhaustion and boost your energy-

- **Protecting your health:** When you ignore your well being, you compromise with your immune system. Dark colored foods that are high on antioxidants like broccoli or berries are the ideal choice to prevent your body from malfunctioning. Also, powdered supplements like Emergen-C can be added to water to bolster your immunity and boost energy.
- **Quit smoking:** If you are a smoker and usually find yourself out of breath post climbing a couple of stairs, no one can understand this better than you. Cigarettes are energy killers which is why typically smokers tend to have lower energy level than non-smokers. The science of this process is rooted in the fact that human body needs to blend oxygen with glucose in order to release energy. On the other hand, cigarettes release carbon monoxide, leaving no room for the blood to absorb oxygen. So whether it's by joining a rehab centre, or by using nicotine patches, stay away from those little killer-dudes!
- **Engage in physical activities:** While physical activity guns down fatigue more efficiently than any other medicine, sedentary lifestyle has been known to be a common cause. A significant bout of exercise not only lures sleep, but also ups your energy levels by creating an adrenaline rush.

- **Leave that desk:** Hogging on a sandwich in front of your computer desk increases the odds of overeating. Get away from your desk to refocus and reenergize yourself at lunchtime.
- **Mind your posture:** Slouching against the chair over your computer can trigger than fatigue-causing hormones earlier than usual. Balance your body weight, sit straight- eyes ahead, shoulder back, with lower back moderately arched. Say no to sloppy postures and get a hike in self confidence.
- **Carpooling:** Feeling dead tired? Not in the mood to catch a bus or other public transport? Well it's better to sleep through your way to the office on the bus rather than finding yourself passed out on your desk.
- **Sun bathing:** A fun fact: Vitamin B and Vitamin D are known to be natural fatigue fighting weapons. Also, Vitamin D is rarely found except in green chilies and sun. Since Vitamin D deficiency might be the cause of tiredness, moodiness and stress, step out in sunshine and give you a 'sunny' treatment for 15 minutes.
- **Turn that cranky switch off:** It is common for fatigue- struck people to feel ready for a confrontation session with those who disturbed them when they were feeling dead on their feet. Psychologists suggest that trying to resist your

cranky urges and turning them off is the first step to a mind-control training program. Be the master of your mind, instead of letting it control you.

- **Communicate, don't connect:** According to several studies conducted over the years, it is self evident how technology has rendered youngsters immobile. You get a new tablet, spend time exploring it, and spend some more time playing with it, and some more. To avoid a sedentary life, go out, hang around with your friends, communicate with your relatives, forget that internet connection and stay active!

- **Pop a gum:** Chewing gums are not known to refresh the breath, but they also revitalize human body quite efficiently. A study conducted in UK in 2012 revealed that those who chewed gum for a few minutes a day showed more signs of alertness than those who did not. Chewing gums boost heart rate, increasing blood flow to your brain and stimulating autonomic nerve system to create alertness.

- **Go 'light' on you:** There's a reason why slumber time and darkness go side by side. Bright light stimulates your senses and awakens the brain. However, not all rays work wonders on our brain. In a study conducted by LRC, New York in 2013, it was found that the strongest midday wakeup call is red light. Surround yourself with red bulbs for an edgy alertness and with blue ones if you prefer a calm alertness.

- **Switch tasks:** It's a workday and the clock strikes 3 p.m. How to beat that afternoon slump? Michigan University studied the typical strategies to overcome a gloomy day and drooping energy levels. The list included switching tasks, designing to-do lists and checking mails on the top. However, these tactics were just not enough to bolster energy and refresh the senses. What worked was engaging the self into learning new things and playing brain games. Fatigue management specialists assert that the more engaging an activity is, the more alert your brain gets.

- **Belt out those rocking songs:** Ever wondered why cranking up your radio makes you push the car accelerator and drive faster? The reason is simple, music is exhilarating. Bob your head, sing your favorite out loud and witness an energy arousal akin to a workout.

- **Give yourself a candy treat:** To be specific, chocolates are known to provide our body with an endorphin buzz (needless to mention the boost of energy we get from a bit of caffeine contained in chocolates). And let's not forget there's a little child in each one of us- who wouldn't love a chocolate in the middle of a day?

- **Wear bright clothes-** While that little hypnotizing black dress might make you feel sexy and confident, psychologists have explored the hidden meaning behind those hues. Red stimulates breathing, blue is for calming that emotional turmoil, yellow speeds up metabolism and green soothes up the senses.

Psychological means of treating fatigue

Studies prove that more than half of the time you feel worn out, the cause is not really fatigue. Rather, it's just your brain tricking you into thinking so. So let those blues fade away by incorporating these simple-to-follow techniques in your routine-

- **Lifestyle assessment:** Are you subjecting yourself to supererogatory stress? Are there any current issues that might be keeping you up late at night and causing anxiety? Ask yourself questions, explore your inner self and assess your lifestyle. If nothing helps, seek expert counseling to solve family and personal issues.

- **Relaxation training:** Constant anxiety can be a really frightening ogre as it drains the entire energy from the body and causes burnouts. One of the most efficient strategies for controlling anxiety is to opt for training in relaxation techniques like yoga, meditation, "switching off" your adrenaline button and allowing the mind to recover.

- **Doing nothing:** One of the major drawbacks of modernization and competitive life is the constant urge to drive oneself to better and bigger heights. A frantic lifestyle is not only exhilarating but also exhausting. Try carving out a couple of hours a day to relax, pamper yourself and hang around doing nothing. Rethink your commitments and priorities.

- **Have fun:** As the famous saying goes- "All work and no play makes Jack a dull boy", having fun is paramount for a working person. So what you have preoccupations or commitments; if you can't find time for yourself, it's just not worth it!

So dodge those midday slumps, lock that frustration in bars and unleash an entirely new level of energy by following these unmistakable tips. Like they say- life's short, laugh out loud and live it to the brim!

www.ingramcontent.com/pod-product-compliance
Lightning Source LLC
Chambersburg PA
CBHW061952280526
45787CB00004B/1831